This Book Belongs To:

_____

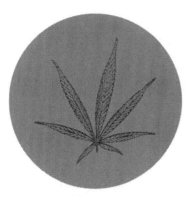

Greatest Hits

Strain:_____   Page #:_____

Strain:_____   Page #:_____

Strain:_____   Page #:_____

Strain:_____   Page #:_____

Strain:_____   Page #:_____

Strain:_____   Page #:_____

Strain:_____   Page #:_____

Strain:_____   Page #:_____

Strain:_____   Page #:_____

Strain:_____   Page #:_____

Strain:_____   Page #:_____

Strain:_____   Page #:_____

Strain:_____   Page #:_____

Strain:_____   Page #:_____

Strain:_____   Page #:_____

Strain:_____   Page #:_____

Strain:_____ Page #:_____

Strain:_____ Page #:_____

Strain:_____ Page #:_____

Strain:_____ Page #:_____

Strain:_____ Page #:_____

Strain:_____ Page #:_____

Strain:_____ Page #:_____

Strain:_____ Page #:_____

Strain:_____ Page #:_____

Strain:_____ Page #:_____

Strain:_____ Page #:_____

Strain:_____ Page #:_____

Strain:_____ Page #:_____

Strain:_____ Page #:_____

Strain:_____ Page #:_____

Strain:_____ Page #:_____

Strain:_____ Page #:_____

Strain:_____ Page #:_____

"I find it quite ironic that the most dangerous things about weed is getting caught with it."

~ Bill Murray

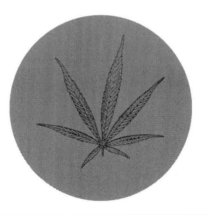

Product

Brand:_____

Name/ Strain:_____

Purchased From:_____

Price:_____

Date Consumed:_____

Current Location:_____

Mood Before Consumption:_____

Mood After Consumption:_____

Product Type	☐ Flower	☐ Edible	☐ Tincture	☐ Topical
	☐ Butter/ Oil	☐ Concentration	☐ Other	

Type	☐ Sativa	☐ Indica	☐ Hybrid

Terpenes	☐ Pinene	☐ Myrcene	☐ Beta- Caryophyllene
	☐ Limonene	☐ Linalool	☐ Terpinolene
	☐ Humulene	☐ Other	

Potency mg or %	THC	CBD	CBN	THCA	Other
	_____	_____	_____	_____	_____

Method

☐ Smoke	☐ Vaporize	☐ Vape Pen	☐ Edible
☐ Drink	☐ Sublingual	☐ Capsule	☐ Patch

Device:_____

Dose/ # Hits:_____

Taste:_____

My Intent:_____

My Experience

Time Consumed:_____ Time to Kick In:_____

Lasted:_____ Strength: 1 2 3 4 5 6 7 8 9 10

Felt it: Head____% Body____% Consume Again: Yes / No

Positive Effects

- Pain Relief
- Stress Reduction
- Anti-Inflammatory
- Energetic

- Muscle Relaxation
- Intestinal Ease
- Creative
- Focused

- Sedative
- Appetite Stimulation
- Anti-Depressant
- Other:

Negative Effects

- Dry Eyes
- Paranoid
- Lethargy

- Anxiety
- Nausea
- Dizziness

- Dry Mouth
- Headache
- Memory Loss

- Confusion
- Drowsy
- Other

Notes

Recommended By:

Recommend To:

Overall Rating:

☆☆☆☆☆

Product

Brand:_____

Name/ Strain:_____

Purchased From:_____

Price:_____

Date Consumed:_____

Current Location:_____

Mood Before Consumption:_____

Mood After Consumption:_____

Product Type	☐ Flower ☐ Butter/ Oil	☐ Edible ☐ Concentration	☐ Tincture ☐ Other	☐ Topical

Type	☐ Sativa	☐ Indica	☐ Hybrid

Terpenes	☐ Pinene ☐ Limonene ☐ Humulene	☐ Myrcene ☐ Linalool ☐ Other	☐ Beta- Caryophyllene ☐ Terpinolene

Potency mg or %	THC	CBD	CBN	THCA	Other
	_____	_____	_____	_____	_____

Method

☐ Smoke	☐ Vaporize	☐ Vape Pen	☐ Edible
☐ Drink	☐ Sublingual	☐ Capsule	☐ Patch

Device:_____

Dose/ # Hits:_____

Taste:_____

My Intent:_____

My Experience

Time Consumed:_____   Time to Kick In:_____
Lasted:_____   Strength: 1 2 3 4 5 6 7 8 9 10
Felt it: Head____% Body____%   Consume Again: Yes / No

Positive Effects

- Pain Relief
- Stress Reduction
- Anti-Inflammatory
- Energetic

- Muscle Relaxation
- Intestinal Ease
- Creative
- Focused

- Sedative
- Appetite Stimulation
- Anti-Depressant
- Other:

Negative Effects

- Dry Eyes
- Paranoid
- Lethargy

- Anxiety
- Nausea
- Dizziness

- Dry Mouth
- Headache
- Memory Loss

- Confusion
- Drowsy
- Other

Notes

Recommended By: Overall Rating:

Recommend To: ☆ ☆ ☆ ☆ ☆

Product

Brand:_____

Name/ Strain:_____

Purchased From:_____

Price:_____

Date Consumed:_____

Current Location:_____

Mood Before Consumption:_____

Mood After Consumption:_____

Product Type	☐ Flower	☐ Edible	☐ Tincture	☐ Topical
	☐ Butter/ Oil	☐ Concentration	☐ Other	

Type	☐ Sativa	☐ Indica	☐ Hybrid

Terpenes	☐ Pinene	☐ Myrcene	☐ Beta- Caryophyllene
	☐ Limonene	☐ Linalool	☐ Terpinolene
	☐ Humulene	☐ Other	

Potency mg or %	THC	CBD	CBN	THCA	Other
	_____	_____	_____	_____	_____

Method

☐ Smoke	☐ Vaporize	☐ Vape Pen	☐ Edible
☐ Drink	☐ Sublingual	☐ Capsule	☐ Patch

Device:_____

Dose/ # Hits:_____

Taste:_____

My Intent:_____

My Experience

Time Consumed:_____   Time to Kick In:_____

Lasted:_____   Strength: 1 2 3 4 5 6 7 8 9 10

Felt it: Head____%   Body____%   Consume Again: Yes / No

Positive Effects

- ☐ Pain Relief
- ☐ Stress Reduction
- ☐ Anti-Inflammatory
- ☐ Energetic
- ☐ Muscle Relaxation
- ☐ Intestinal Ease
- ☐ Creative
- ☐ Focused
- ☐ Sedative
- ☐ Appetite Stimulation
- ☐ Anti-Depressant
- ☐ Other:

Negative Effects

- ☐ Dry Eyes
- ☐ Paranoid
- ☐ Lethargy
- ☐ Anxiety
- ☐ Nausea
- ☐ Dizziness
- ☐ Dry Mouth
- ☐ Headache
- ☐ Memory Loss
- ☐ Confusion
- ☐ Drowsy
- ☐ Other

Notes

_____
_____
_____
_____
_____
_____
_____

Recommended By: _____

Recommend To: _____

Overall Rating:

☆ ☆ ☆ ☆ ☆

Product

Brand:_____

Name/ Strain:_____

Purchased From:_____

Price:_____

Date Consumed:_____

Current Location:_____

Mood Before Consumption:_____

Mood After Consumption:_____

Product Type	☐ Flower ☐ Butter/ Oil	☐ Edible ☐ Concentration	☐ Tincture ☐ Other	☐ Topical

Type	☐ Sativa	☐ Indica	☐ Hybrid

Terpenes	☐ Pinene ☐ Limonene ☐ Humulene	☐ Myrcene ☐ Linalool ☐ Other	☐ Beta- Caryophyllene ☐ Terpinolene

Potency mg or %	THC	CBD	CBN	THCA	Other
	_____	_____	_____	_____	_____

Method

☐ Smoke	☐ Vaporize	☐ Vape Pen	☐ Edible
☐ Drink	☐ Sublingual	☐ Capsule	☐ Patch

Device:_____

Dose/ # Hits:_____

Taste:_____

My Intent:_____

My Experience

Time Consumed:_____   Time to Kick In:_____
Lasted:_____   Strength: 1 2 3 4 5 6 7 8 9 10
Felt it: Head____% Body____%   Consume Again: Yes / No

Positive Effects

- [ ] Pain Relief
- [ ] Stress Reduction
- [ ] Anti-Inflammatory
- [ ] Energetic
- [ ] Muscle Relaxation
- [ ] Intestinal Ease
- [ ] Creative
- [ ] Focused
- [ ] Sedative
- [ ] Appetite Stimulation
- [ ] Anti-Depressant
- [ ] Other:

Negative Effects

- [ ] Dry Eyes
- [ ] Paranoid
- [ ] Lethargy
- [ ] Anxiety
- [ ] Nausea
- [ ] Dizziness
- [ ] Dry Mouth
- [ ] Headache
- [ ] Memory Loss
- [ ] Confusion
- [ ] Drowsy
- [ ] Other

Notes

Recommended By:

Recommend To:

Overall Rating:

☆ ☆ ☆ ☆ ☆

Product

Brand:_____

Name/ Strain:_____

Purchased From:_____

Price:_____

Date Consumed:_____

Current Location:_____

Mood Before Consumption:_____

Mood After Consumption:_____

Product Type	☐ Flower ☐ Butter/ Oil	☐ Edible ☐ Concentration	☐ Tincture ☐ Other	☐ Topical

Type	☐ Sativa	☐ Indica	☐ Hybrid

Terpenes	☐ Pinene ☐ Limonene ☐ Humulene	☐ Myrcene ☐ Linalool ☐ Other	☐ Beta- Caryophyllene ☐ Terpinolene

Potency mg or %	THC	CBD	CBN	THCA	Other
	_____	_____	_____	_____	_____

Method

☐ Smoke ☐ Vaporize ☐ Vape Pen ☐ Edible
☐ Drink ☐ Sublingual ☐ Capsule ☐ Patch

Device:_____

Dose/ # Hits:_____

Taste:_____

My Intent:_____

My Experience

Time Consumed:_____   Time to Kick In:_____

Lasted:_____   Strength: 1 2 3 4 5 6 7 8 9 10

Felt it: Head___% Body___%   Consume Again: Yes / No

Positive Effects

- Pain Relief
- Stress Reduction
- Anti-Inflammatory
- Energetic

- Muscle Relaxation
- Intestinal Ease
- Creative
- Focused

- Sedative
- Appetite Stimulation
- Anti-Depressant
- Other:

Negative Effects

- Dry Eyes
- Paranoid
- Lethargy

- Anxiety
- Nausea
- Dizziness

- Dry Mouth
- Headache
- Memory Loss

- Confusion
- Drowsy
- Other

Notes

Recommended By:

Recommend To:

Overall Rating:

☆ ☆ ☆ ☆ ☆

Product

Brand:_____

Name/ Strain:_____

Purchased From:_____

Price:_____

Date Consumed:_____

Current Location:_____

Mood Before Consumption:_____

Mood After Consumption:_____

Product Type	☐ Flower ☐ Butter/ Oil	☐ Edible ☐ Concentration	☐ Tincture ☐ Other	☐ Topical

Type	☐ Sativa	☐ Indica	☐ Hybrid

Terpenes	☐ Pinene ☐ Limonene ☐ Humulene	☐ Myrcene ☐ Linalool ☐ Other	☐ Beta- Caryophyllene ☐ Terpinolene

Potency mg or %	THC	CBD	CBN	THCA	Other
	_____	_____	_____	_____	_____

Method

☐ Smoke	☐ Vaporize	☐ Vape Pen	☐ Edible
☐ Drink	☐ Sublingual	☐ Capsule	☐ Patch

Device:_____

Dose/ # Hits:_____

Taste:_____

My Intent:_____

My Experience

Time Consumed:_____   Time to Kick In:_____
Lasted:_____   Strength: 1 2 3 4 5 6 7 8 9 10
Felt it: Head____%   Body____%   Consume Again: Yes / No

Positive Effects

- ☐ Pain Relief
- ☐ Stress Reduction
- ☐ Anti-Inflammatory
- ☐ Energetic
- ☐ Muscle Relaxation
- ☐ Intestinal Ease
- ☐ Creative
- ☐ Focused
- ☐ Sedative
- ☐ Appetite Stimulation
- ☐ Anti-Depressant
- ☐ Other:

Negative Effects

- ☐ Dry Eyes
- ☐ Paranoid
- ☐ Lethargy
- ☐ Anxiety
- ☐ Nausea
- ☐ Dizziness
- ☐ Dry Mouth
- ☐ Headache
- ☐ Memory Loss
- ☐ Confusion
- ☐ Drowsy
- ☐ Other

Notes

Recommended By:

Recommend To:

Overall Rating:

☆ ☆ ☆ ☆ ☆

Product

Brand:_____

Name/ Strain:_____

Purchased From:_____

Price:_____

Date Consumed:_____

Current Location:_____

Mood Before Consumption:_____

Mood After Consumption:_____

| **Product Type** | ☐ Flower | ☐ Edible | ☐ Tincture | ☐ Topical |
| | ☐ Butter/ Oil | ☐ Concentration | ☐ Other | |

| **Type** | ☐ Sativa | ☐ Indica | ☐ Hybrid |

Terpenes	☐ Pinene	☐ Myrcene	☐ Beta- Caryophyllene
	☐ Limonene	☐ Linalool	☐ Terpinolene
	☐ Humulene	☐ Other	

| **Potency mg or %** | THC | CBD | CBN | THCA | Other |
| | _____ | _____ | _____ | _____ | _____ |

Method

| ☐ Smoke | ☐ Vaporize | ☐ Vape Pen | ☐ Edible |
| ☐ Drink | ☐ Sublingual | ☐ Capsule | ☐ Patch |

Device:_____

Dose/ # Hits:_____

Taste:_____

My Intent:_____

My Experience

Time Consumed:_____   Time to Kick In:_____

Lasted:_____   Strength: 1 2 3 4 5 6 7 8 9 10

Felt it: Head____% Body____%   Consume Again: Yes / No

Positive Effects

- ☐ Pain Relief
- ☐ Stress Reduction
- ☐ Anti-Inflammatory
- ☐ Energetic

- ☐ Muscle Relaxation
- ☐ Intestinal Ease
- ☐ Creative
- ☐ Focused

- ☐ Sedative
- ☐ Appetite Stimulation
- ☐ Anti-Depressant
- ☐ Other:

Negative Effects

- ☐ Dry Eyes
- ☐ Paranoid
- ☐ Lethargy

- ☐ Anxiety
- ☐ Nausea
- ☐ Dizziness

- ☐ Dry Mouth
- ☐ Headache
- ☐ Memory Loss

- ☐ Confusion
- ☐ Drowsy
- ☐ Other

Notes

Recommended By:_____

Recommend To:_____

Overall Rating:

☆ ☆ ☆ ☆ ☆

Product

Brand:_____

Name/ Strain:_____

Purchased From:_____

Price:_____

Date Consumed:_____

Current Location:_____

Mood Before Consumption:_____

Mood After Consumption:_____

Product Type	☐ Flower ☐ Butter/ Oil	☐ Edible ☐ Concentration	☐ Tincture ☐ Other	☐ Topical

Type	☐ Sativa	☐ Indica	☐ Hybrid

Terpenes	☐ Pinene ☐ Limonene ☐ Humulene	☐ Myrcene ☐ Linalool ☐ Other	☐ Beta- Caryophyllene ☐ Terpinolene

Potency mg or %	THC	CBD	CBN	THCA	Other
	_____	_____	_____	_____	_____

Method

☐ Smoke	☐ Vaporize	☐ Vape Pen	☐ Edible
☐ Drink	☐ Sublingual	☐ Capsule	☐ Patch

Device:_____

Dose/ # Hits:_____

Taste:_____

My Intent:_____

My Experience

Time Consumed:_____   Time to Kick In:_____

Lasted:_____   Strength: 1 2 3 4 5 6 7 8 9 10

Felt it: Head____%   Body____%   Consume Again: Yes / No

Positive Effects

- ☐ Pain Relief
- ☐ Stress Reduction
- ☐ Anti-Inflammatory
- ☐ Energetic

- ☐ Muscle Relaxation
- ☐ Intestinal Ease
- ☐ Creative
- ☐ Focused

- ☐ Sedative
- ☐ Appetite Stimulation
- ☐ Anti-Depressant
- ☐ Other:

Negative Effects

- ☐ Dry Eyes
- ☐ Paranoid
- ☐ Lethargy

- ☐ Anxiety
- ☐ Nausea
- ☐ Dizziness

- ☐ Dry Mouth
- ☐ Headache
- ☐ Memory Loss

- ☐ Confusion
- ☐ Drowsy
- ☐ Other

Notes

Recommended By:

Recommend To:

Overall Rating:

☆ ☆ ☆ ☆ ☆

Product

Brand:_____

Name/ Strain:_____

Purchased From:_____

Price:_____

Date Consumed:_____

Current Location:_____

Mood Before Consumption:_____

Mood After Consumption:_____

Product Type	☐ Flower ☐ Butter/ Oil	☐ Edible ☐ Concentration	☐ Tincture ☐ Other	☐ Topical

Type	☐ Sativa	☐ Indica	☐ Hybrid

Terpenes	☐ Pinene ☐ Limonene ☐ Humulene	☐ Myrcene ☐ Linalool ☐ Other	☐ Beta- Caryophyllene ☐ Terpinolene

Potency mg or %	THC	CBD	CBN	THCA	Other
	_____	_____	_____	_____	_____

Method

☐ Smoke   ☐ Vaporize   ☐ Vape Pen   ☐ Edible
☐ Drink   ☐ Sublingual   ☐ Capsule   ☐ Patch

Device:_____

Dose/ # Hits:_____

Taste:_____

My Intent:_____

My Experience

Time Consumed:_____   Time to Kick In:_____

Lasted:_____   Strength: 1 2 3 4 5 6 7 8 9 10

Felt it: Head____% Body____%   Consume Again: Yes / No

Positive Effects

- [ ] Pain Relief
- [ ] Stress Reduction
- [ ] Anti-Inflammatory
- [ ] Energetic
- [ ] Muscle Relaxation
- [ ] Intestinal Ease
- [ ] Creative
- [ ] Focused
- [ ] Sedative
- [ ] Appetite Stimulation
- [ ] Anti-Depressant
- [ ] Other:

Negative Effects

- [ ] Dry Eyes
- [ ] Paranoid
- [ ] Lethargy
- [ ] Anxiety
- [ ] Nausea
- [ ] Dizziness
- [ ] Dry Mouth
- [ ] Headache
- [ ] Memory Loss
- [ ] Confusion
- [ ] Drowsy
- [ ] Other

Notes

Recommended By: _____

Recommend To: _____

Overall Rating:

☆ ☆ ☆ ☆ ☆

Product

Brand:_____

Name/ Strain:_____

Purchased From:_____

Price:_____

Date Consumed:_____

Current Location:_____

Mood Before Consumption:_____

Mood After Consumption:_____

Product Type	☐ Flower ☐ Butter/ Oil	☐ Edible ☐ Concentration	☐ Tincture ☐ Other	☐ Topical

Type	☐ Sativa	☐ Indica	☐ Hybrid

Terpenes	☐ Pinene ☐ Limonene ☐ Humulene	☐ Myrcene ☐ Linalool ☐ Other	☐ Beta- Caryophyllene ☐ Terpinolene

Potency mg or %	THC	CBD	CBN	THCA	Other
	_____	_____	_____	_____	_____

Method

☐ Smoke ☐ Vaporize ☐ Vape Pen ☐ Edible
☐ Drink ☐ Sublingual ☐ Capsule ☐ Patch

Device:_____

Dose/ # Hits:_____

Taste:_____

My Intent:_____

My Experience

Time Consumed:_____   Time to Kick In:_____
Lasted:_____   Strength: 1 2 3 4 5 6 7 8 9 10
Felt it: Head____%   Body____%   Consume Again: Yes / No

Positive Effects

☐ Pain Relief   ☐ Muscle Relaxation   ☐ Sedative
☐ Stress Reduction   ☐ Intestinal Ease   ☐ Appetite Stimulation
☐ Anti-Inflammatory   ☐ Creative   ☐ Anti-Depressant
☐ Energetic   ☐ Focused   ☐ Other:

Negative Effects

☐ Dry Eyes   ☐ Anxiety   ☐ Dry Mouth   ☐ Confusion
☐ Paranoid   ☐ Nausea   ☐ Headache   ☐ Drowsy
☐ Lethargy   ☐ Dizziness   ☐ Memory Loss   ☐ Other

Notes

Recommended By: Overall Rating:

Recommend To: ☆ ☆ ☆ ☆ ☆

Product

Brand:_____

Name/ Strain:_____

Purchased From:_____

Price:_____

Date Consumed:_____

Current Location:_____

Mood Before Consumption:_____

Mood After Consumption:_____

| Product Type | ☐ Flower | ☐ Edible | ☐ Tincture | ☐ Topical |
| | ☐ Butter/ Oil | ☐ Concentration | ☐ Other | |

| Type | ☐ Sativa | ☐ Indica | ☐ Hybrid |

Terpenes	☐ Pinene	☐ Myrcene	☐ Beta- Caryophyllene
	☐ Limonene	☐ Linalool	☐ Terpinolene
	☐ Humulene	☐ Other	

| Potency mg or % | THC | CBD | CBN | THCA | Other |
| | _____ | _____ | _____ | _____ | _____ |

Method

| ☐ Smoke | ☐ Vaporize | ☐ Vape Pen | ☐ Edible |
| ☐ Drink | ☐ Sublingual | ☐ Capsule | ☐ Patch |

Device:_____

Dose/ # Hits:_____

Taste:_____

My Intent:_____

My Experience

Time Consumed:_____   Time to Kick In:_____
Lasted:_____   Strength: 1 2 3 4 5 6 7 8 9 10
Felt it: Head___% Body___%   Consume Again: Yes / No

Positive Effects

- Pain Relief
- Stress Reduction
- Anti-Inflammatory
- Energetic

- Muscle Relaxation
- Intestinal Ease
- Creative
- Focused

- Sedative
- Appetite Stimulation
- Anti-Depressant
- Other:

Negative Effects

- Dry Eyes
- Paranoid
- Lethargy

- Anxiety
- Nausea
- Dizziness

- Dry Mouth
- Headache
- Memory Loss

- Confusion
- Drowsy
- Other

Notes

Recommended By:

Recommend To:

Overall Rating:

☆ ☆ ☆ ☆ ☆

Product

Brand:_____

Name/ Strain:_____

Purchased From:_____

Price:_____

Date Consumed:_____

Current Location:_____

Mood Before Consumption:_____

Mood After Consumption:_____

Product Type	☐ Flower ☐ Butter/ Oil	☐ Edible ☐ Concentration	☐ Tincture ☐ Other	☐ Topical

Type	☐ Sativa	☐ Indica	☐ Hybrid

Terpenes	☐ Pinene ☐ Limonene ☐ Humulene	☐ Myrcene ☐ Linalool ☐ Other	☐ Beta- Caryophyllene ☐ Terpinolene

Potency mg or %	THC	CBD	CBN	THCA	Other
	_____	_____	_____	_____	_____

Method

☐ Smoke   ☐ Vaporize   ☐ Vape Pen   ☐ Edible
☐ Drink   ☐ Sublingual   ☐ Capsule   ☐ Patch

Device:_____

Dose/ # Hits:_____

Taste:_____

My Intent:_____

My Experience

Time Consumed:_____   Time to Kick In:_____
Lasted:_____   Strength: 1 2 3 4 5 6 7 8 9 10
Felt it: Head____%   Body____%   Consume Again: Yes / No

Positive Effects

- ☐ Pain Relief
- ☐ Stress Reduction
- ☐ Anti-Inflammatory
- ☐ Energetic
- ☐ Muscle Relaxation
- ☐ Intestinal Ease
- ☐ Creative
- ☐ Focused
- ☐ Sedative
- ☐ Appetite Stimulation
- ☐ Anti-Depressant
- ☐ Other:

Negative Effects

- ☐ Dry Eyes
- ☐ Paranoid
- ☐ Lethargy
- ☐ Anxiety
- ☐ Nausea
- ☐ Dizziness
- ☐ Dry Mouth
- ☐ Headache
- ☐ Memory Loss
- ☐ Confusion
- ☐ Drowsy
- ☐ Other

Notes

Recommended By:_____

Recommend To:_____

Overall Rating:

☆ ☆ ☆ ☆ ☆

Product

Brand:_____

Name/ Strain:_____

Purchased From:_____

Price:_____

Date Consumed:_____

Current Location:_____

Mood Before Consumption:_____

Mood After Consumption:_____

Product Type	☐ Flower	☐ Edible	☐ Tincture	☐ Topical
	☐ Butter/ Oil	☐ Concentration	☐ Other	

Type	☐ Sativa	☐ Indica	☐ Hybrid

Terpenes	☐ Pinene	☐ Myrcene	☐ Beta- Caryophyllene
	☐ Limonene	☐ Linalool	☐ Terpinolene
	☐ Humulene	☐ Other	

Potency mg or %	THC	CBD	CBN	THCA	Other
	_____	_____	_____	_____	_____

Method

☐ Smoke	☐ Vaporize	☐ Vape Pen	☐ Edible
☐ Drink	☐ Sublingual	☐ Capsule	☐ Patch

Device:_____

Dose/ # Hits:_____

Taste:_____

My Intent:_____

My Experience

Time Consumed:_____   Time to Kick In:_____

Lasted:_____   Strength: 1 2 3 4 5 6 7 8 9 10

Felt it: Head____%   Body____%   Consume Again: Yes / No

Positive Effects

- ☐ Pain Relief
- ☐ Stress Reduction
- ☐ Anti-Inflammatory
- ☐ Energetic

- ☐ Muscle Relaxation
- ☐ Intestinal Ease
- ☐ Creative
- ☐ Focused

- ☐ Sedative
- ☐ Appetite Stimulation
- ☐ Anti-Depressant
- ☐ Other:

Negative Effects

- ☐ Dry Eyes
- ☐ Paranoid
- ☐ Lethargy

- ☐ Anxiety
- ☐ Nausea
- ☐ Dizziness

- ☐ Dry Mouth
- ☐ Headache
- ☐ Memory Loss

- ☐ Confusion
- ☐ Drowsy
- ☐ Other

Notes

Recommended By:_____

Recommend To:_____

Overall Rating:

☆ ☆ ☆ ☆ ☆

Product

Brand:_____

Name/ Strain:_____

Purchased From:_____

Price:_____

Date Consumed:_____

Current Location:_____

Mood Before Consumption:_____

Mood After Consumption:_____

Product Type	☐ Flower	☐ Edible	☐ Tincture	☐ Topical
	☐ Butter/ Oil	☐ Concentration	☐ Other	

Type	☐ Sativa	☐ Indica	☐ Hybrid

Terpenes	☐ Pinene	☐ Myrcene	☐ Beta- Caryophyllene
	☐ Limonene	☐ Linalool	☐ Terpinolene
	☐ Humulene	☐ Other	

Potency mg or %	THC	CBD	CBN	THCA	Other
	_____	_____	_____	_____	_____

Method

☐ Smoke	☐ Vaporize	☐ Vape Pen	☐ Edible
☐ Drink	☐ Sublingual	☐ Capsule	☐ Patch

Device:_____

Dose/ # Hits:_____

Taste:_____

My Intent:_____

My Experience

Time Consumed:_____   Time to Kick In:_____

Lasted:_____   Strength: 1 2 3 4 5 6 7 8 9 10

Felt it: Head____%   Body____%   Consume Again: Yes / No

Positive Effects

- ☐ Pain Relief
- ☐ Stress Reduction
- ☐ Anti-Inflammatory
- ☐ Energetic
- ☐ Muscle Relaxation
- ☐ Intestinal Ease
- ☐ Creative
- ☐ Focused
- ☐ Sedative
- ☐ Appetite Stimulation
- ☐ Anti-Depressant
- ☐ Other:

Negative Effects

- ☐ Dry Eyes
- ☐ Paranoid
- ☐ Lethargy
- ☐ Anxiety
- ☐ Nausea
- ☐ Dizziness
- ☐ Dry Mouth
- ☐ Headache
- ☐ Memory Loss
- ☐ Confusion
- ☐ Drowsy
- ☐ Other

Notes

Recommended By:

Recommend To:

Overall Rating:

☆ ☆ ☆ ☆ ☆

Product

Brand:_____

Name/ Strain:_____

Purchased From:_____

Price:_____

Date Consumed:_____

Current Location:_____

Mood Before Consumption:_____

Mood After Consumption:_____

Product Type	☐ Flower ☐ Butter/ Oil	☐ Edible ☐ Concentration	☐ Tincture ☐ Other	☐ Topical

Type	☐ Sativa	☐ Indica	☐ Hybrid

Terpenes	☐ Pinene ☐ Limonene ☐ Humulene	☐ Myrcene ☐ Linalool ☐ Other	☐ Beta- Caryophyllene ☐ Terpinolene

Potency mg or %	THC	CBD	CBN	THCA	Other
	_____	_____	_____	_____	_____

Method

☐ Smoke   ☐ Vaporize   ☐ Vape Pen   ☐ Edible
☐ Drink   ☐ Sublingual   ☐ Capsule   ☐ Patch

Device:_____

Dose/ # Hits:_____

Taste:_____

My Intent:_____

My Experience

Time Consumed:_____   Time to Kick In:_____
Lasted:_____   Strength: 1 2 3 4 5 6 7 8 9 10
Felt it: Head____%   Body____% Consume Again: Yes / No

Positive Effects

☐ Pain Relief   ☐ Muscle Relaxation   ☐ Sedative
☐ Stress Reduction   ☐ Intestinal Ease   ☐ Appetite Stimulation
☐ Anti-Inflammatory   ☐ Creative   ☐ Anti-Depressant
☐ Energetic   ☐ Focused   ☐ Other:

Negative Effects

☐ Dry Eyes   ☐ Anxiety   ☐ Dry Mouth   ☐ Confusion
☐ Paranoid   ☐ Nausea   ☐ Headache   ☐ Drowsy
☐ Lethargy   ☐ Dizziness   ☐ Memory Loss   ☐ Other

Notes

Recommended By: Overall Rating:
_____   ☆ ☆ ☆ ☆ ☆
Recommend To:
_____

Product

Brand:_____

Name/ Strain:_____

Purchased From:_____

Price:_____

Date Consumed:_____

Current Location:_____

Mood Before Consumption:_____

Mood After Consumption:_____

Product Type	☐ Flower ☐ Butter/ Oil	☐ Edible ☐ Concentration	☐ Tincture ☐ Other	☐ Topical

Type	☐ Sativa	☐ Indica	☐ Hybrid

Terpenes	☐ Pinene ☐ Limonene ☐ Humulene	☐ Myrcene ☐ Linalool ☐ Other	☐ Beta- Caryophyllene ☐ Terpinolene

Potency mg or %	THC	CBD	CBN	THCA	Other
	_____	_____	_____	_____	_____

Method

☐ Smoke   ☐ Vaporize   ☐ Vape Pen   ☐ Edible
☐ Drink   ☐ Sublingual   ☐ Capsule   ☐ Patch

Device:_____

Dose/ # Hits:_____

Taste:_____

My Intent:_____

My Experience

Time Consumed:_____   Time to Kick In:_____
Lasted:_____   Strength: 1 2 3 4 5 6 7 8 9 10
Felt it: Head___% Body___%   Consume Again: Yes / No

Positive Effects

☐ Pain Relief   ☐ Muscle Relaxation   ☐ Sedative
☐ Stress Reduction   ☐ Intestinal Ease   ☐ Appetite Stimulation
☐ Anti-Inflammatory   ☐ Creative   ☐ Anti-Depressant
☐ Energetic   ☐ Focused   ☐ Other:

Negative Effects

☐ Dry Eyes   ☐ Anxiety   ☐ Dry Mouth   ☐ Confusion
☐ Paranoid   ☐ Nausea   ☐ Headache   ☐ Drowsy
☐ Lethargy   ☐ Dizziness   ☐ Memory Loss   ☐ Other

Notes

Recommended By: Overall Rating:

Recommend To: ☆ ☆ ☆ ☆ ☆

Product

Brand:_____

Name/ Strain:_____

Purchased From:_____

Price:_____

Date Consumed:_____

Current Location:_____

Mood Before Consumption:_____

Mood After Consumption:_____

| **Product Type** | ☐ Flower | ☐ Edible | ☐ Tincture | ☐ Topical |
| | ☐ Butter/ Oil | ☐ Concentration | ☐ Other | |

| **Type** | ☐ Sativa | ☐ Indica | ☐ Hybrid |

Terpenes	☐ Pinene	☐ Myrcene	☐ Beta- Caryophyllene
	☐ Limonene	☐ Linalool	☐ Terpinolene
	☐ Humulene	☐ Other	

| **Potency mg or %** | THC | CBD | CBN | THCA | Other |
| | _____ | _____ | _____ | _____ | _____ |

Method

| ☐ Smoke | ☐ Vaporize | ☐ Vape Pen | ☐ Edible |
| ☐ Drink | ☐ Sublingual | ☐ Capsule | ☐ Patch |

Device:_____

Dose/ # Hits:_____

Taste:_____

My Intent:_____

My Experience

Time Consumed:_____ Time to Kick In:_____
Lasted:_____ Strength: 1 2 3 4 5 6 7 8 9 10
Felt it: Head____% Body____% Consume Again: Yes / No

Positive Effects

- ☐ Pain Relief
- ☐ Stress Reduction
- ☐ Anti-Inflammatory
- ☐ Energetic
- ☐ Muscle Relaxation
- ☐ Intestinal Ease
- ☐ Creative
- ☐ Focused
- ☐ Sedative
- ☐ Appetite Stimulation
- ☐ Anti-Depressant
- ☐ Other:

Negative Effects

- ☐ Dry Eyes
- ☐ Paranoid
- ☐ Lethargy
- ☐ Anxiety
- ☐ Nausea
- ☐ Dizziness
- ☐ Dry Mouth
- ☐ Headache
- ☐ Memory Loss
- ☐ Confusion
- ☐ Drowsy
- ☐ Other

Notes

Recommended By:_____

Recommend To:_____

Overall Rating:

☆ ☆ ☆ ☆ ☆

Product

Brand:_____

Name/ Strain:_____

Purchased From:_____

Price:_____

Date Consumed:_____

Current Location:_____

Mood Before Consumption:_____

Mood After Consumption:_____

| **Product Type** | ☐ Flower   ☐ Edible   ☐ Tincture   ☐ Topical |
| | ☐ Butter/ Oil   ☐ Concentration   ☐ Other |

| **Type** | ☐ Sativa | ☐ Indica | ☐ Hybrid |

Terpenes	☐ Pinene ☐ Myrcene ☐ Beta- Caryophyllene
	☐ Limonene ☐ Linalool ☐ Terpinolene
	☐ Humulene ☐ Other

Potency mg or %	THC	CBD	CBN	THCA	Other
	_____	_____	_____	_____	_____

Method

☐ Smoke   ☐ Vaporize   ☐ Vape Pen   ☐ Edible
☐ Drink   ☐ Sublingual   ☐ Capsule   ☐ Patch

Device:_____

Dose/ # Hits:_____

Taste:_____

My Intent:_____

My Experience

Time Consumed:_____   Time to Kick In:_____
Lasted:_____   Strength: 1 2 3 4 5 6 7 8 9 10
Felt it: Head____%   Body____%   Consume Again: Yes / No

Positive Effects

- ☐ Pain Relief
- ☐ Stress Reduction
- ☐ Anti-Inflammatory
- ☐ Energetic
- ☐ Muscle Relaxation
- ☐ Intestinal Ease
- ☐ Creative
- ☐ Focused
- ☐ Sedative
- ☐ Appetite Stimulation
- ☐ Anti-Depressant
- ☐ Other:

Negative Effects

- ☐ Dry Eyes
- ☐ Paranoid
- ☐ Lethargy
- ☐ Anxiety
- ☐ Nausea
- ☐ Dizziness
- ☐ Dry Mouth
- ☐ Headache
- ☐ Memory Loss
- ☐ Confusion
- ☐ Drowsy
- ☐ Other

Notes

Recommended By:_____

Recommend To:_____

Overall Rating:

☆ ☆ ☆ ☆ ☆

Product

Brand:_____

Name/ Strain:_____

Purchased From:_____

Price:_____

Date Consumed:_____

Current Location:_____

Mood Before Consumption:_____

Mood After Consumption:_____

Product Type	☐ Flower ☐ Butter/ Oil	☐ Edible ☐ Concentration	☐ Tincture ☐ Other	☐ Topical

Type	☐ Sativa	☐ Indica	☐ Hybrid

Terpenes	☐ Pinene ☐ Limonene ☐ Humulene	☐ Myrcene ☐ Linalool ☐ Other	☐ Beta- Caryophyllene ☐ Terpinolene

Potency mg or %	THC	CBD	CBN	THCA	Other
	_____	_____	_____	_____	_____

Method

☐ Smoke ☐ Drink	☐ Vaporize ☐ Sublingual	☐ Vape Pen ☐ Capsule	☐ Edible ☐ Patch

Device:_____

Dose/ # Hits:_____

Taste:_____

My Intent:_____

My Experience

Time Consumed:_____   Time to Kick In:_____

Lasted:_____   Strength: 1 2 3 4 5 6 7 8 9 10

Felt it: Head____%   Body____%   Consume Again: Yes / No

Positive Effects

☐ Pain Relief   ☐ Muscle Relaxation   ☐ Sedative
☐ Stress Reduction   ☐ Intestinal Ease   ☐ Appetite Stimulation
☐ Anti-Inflammatory   ☐ Creative   ☐ Anti-Depressant
☐ Energetic   ☐ Focused   ☐ Other:

Negative Effects

☐ Dry Eyes   ☐ Anxiety   ☐ Dry Mouth   ☐ Confusion
☐ Paranoid   ☐ Nausea   ☐ Headache   ☐ Drowsy
☐ Lethargy   ☐ Dizziness   ☐ Memory Loss   ☐ Other

Notes

Recommended By: Overall Rating:

Recommend To: ☆ ☆ ☆ ☆ ☆

Product

Brand:_____

Name/ Strain:_____

Purchased From:_____

Price:_____

Date Consumed:_____

Current Location:_____

Mood Before Consumption:_____

Mood After Consumption:_____

| **Product Type** | ☐ Flower | ☐ Edible | ☐ Tincture | ☐ Topical |
| | ☐ Butter/ Oil | ☐ Concentration | ☐ Other | |

| **Type** | ☐ Sativa | ☐ Indica | ☐ Hybrid |

Terpenes	☐ Pinene	☐ Myrcene	☐ Beta- Caryophyllene
	☐ Limonene	☐ Linalool	☐ Terpinolene
	☐ Humulene	☐ Other	

| **Potency mg or %** | THC | CBD | CBN | THCA | Other |
| | _____ | _____ | _____ | _____ | _____ |

Method

| ☐ Smoke | ☐ Vaporize | ☐ Vape Pen | ☐ Edible |
| ☐ Drink | ☐ Sublingual | ☐ Capsule | ☐ Patch |

Device:_____

Dose/ # Hits:_____

Taste:_____

My Intent:_____

My Experience

Time Consumed:_____   Time to Kick In:_____

Lasted:_____   Strength: 1 2 3 4 5 6 7 8 9 10

Felt it: Head____% Body____%   Consume Again: Yes / No

Positive Effects

- ☐ Pain Relief
- ☐ Stress Reduction
- ☐ Anti-Inflammatory
- ☐ Energetic
- ☐ Muscle Relaxation
- ☐ Intestinal Ease
- ☐ Creative
- ☐ Focused
- ☐ Sedative
- ☐ Appetite Stimulation
- ☐ Anti-Depressant
- ☐ Other:

Negative Effects

- ☐ Dry Eyes
- ☐ Paranoid
- ☐ Lethargy
- ☐ Anxiety
- ☐ Nausea
- ☐ Dizziness
- ☐ Dry Mouth
- ☐ Headache
- ☐ Memory Loss
- ☐ Confusion
- ☐ Drowsy
- ☐ Other

Notes

Recommended By:_____

Recommend To:_____

Overall Rating:

☆ ☆ ☆ ☆ ☆

Product

Brand:_____

Name/ Strain:_____

Purchased From:_____

Price:_____

Date Consumed:_____

Current Location:_____

Mood Before Consumption:_____

Mood After Consumption:_____

Product Type	☐ Flower ☐ Butter/ Oil	☐ Edible ☐ Concentration	☐ Tincture ☐ Other	☐ Topical

Type	☐ Sativa	☐ Indica	☐ Hybrid

Terpenes	☐ Pinene ☐ Limonene ☐ Humulene	☐ Myrcene ☐ Linalool ☐ Other	☐ Beta- Caryophyllene ☐ Terpinolene

Potency mg or %	THC	CBD	CBN	THCA	Other
	_____	_____	_____	_____	_____

Method

☐ Smoke   ☐ Vaporize   ☐ Vape Pen   ☐ Edible
☐ Drink   ☐ Sublingual   ☐ Capsule   ☐ Patch

Device:_____

Dose/ # Hits:_____

Taste:_____

My Intent:_____

My Experience

Time Consumed:_____   Time to Kick In:_____
Lasted:_____   Strength: 1 2 3 4 5 6 7 8 9 10
Felt it: Head____% Body____%   Consume Again: Yes / No

Positive Effects

- ☐ Pain Relief
- ☐ Stress Reduction
- ☐ Anti-Inflammatory
- ☐ Energetic
- ☐ Muscle Relaxation
- ☐ Intestinal Ease
- ☐ Creative
- ☐ Focused
- ☐ Sedative
- ☐ Appetite Stimulation
- ☐ Anti-Depressant
- ☐ Other:

Negative Effects

- ☐ Dry Eyes
- ☐ Paranoid
- ☐ Lethargy
- ☐ Anxiety
- ☐ Nausea
- ☐ Dizziness
- ☐ Dry Mouth
- ☐ Headache
- ☐ Memory Loss
- ☐ Confusion
- ☐ Drowsy
- ☐ Other

Notes

Recommended By:

Recommend To:

Overall Rating:

☆ ☆ ☆ ☆ ☆

Product

Brand:_____

Name/ Strain:_____

Purchased From:_____

Price:_____

Date Consumed:_____

Current Location:_____

Mood Before Consumption:_____

Mood After Consumption:_____

Product Type	☐ Flower ☐ Butter/ Oil	☐ Edible ☐ Concentration	☐ Tincture ☐ Other	☐ Topical

Type	☐ Sativa	☐ Indica	☐ Hybrid

Terpenes	☐ Pinene ☐ Limonene ☐ Humulene	☐ Myrcene ☐ Linalool ☐ Other	☐ Beta- Caryophyllene ☐ Terpinolene

Potency mg or %	THC	CBD	CBN	THCA	Other
	_____	_____	_____	_____	_____

Method

☐ Smoke   ☐ Vaporize   ☐ Vape Pen   ☐ Edible
☐ Drink   ☐ Sublingual   ☐ Capsule   ☐ Patch

Device:_____

Dose/ # Hits:_____

Taste:_____

My Intent:_____

My Experience

Time Consumed:_____   Time to Kick In:_____
Lasted:_____   Strength: 1 2 3 4 5 6 7 8 9 10
Felt it: Head____% Body____%   Consume Again: Yes / No

Positive Effects

☐ Pain Relief   ☐ Muscle Relaxation   ☐ Sedative
☐ Stress Reduction   ☐ Intestinal Ease   ☐ Appetite Stimulation
☐ Anti-Inflammatory   ☐ Creative   ☐ Anti-Depressant
☐ Energetic   ☐ Focused   ☐ Other:

Negative Effects

☐ Dry Eyes   ☐ Anxiety   ☐ Dry Mouth   ☐ Confusion
☐ Paranoid   ☐ Nausea   ☐ Headache   ☐ Drowsy
☐ Lethargy   ☐ Dizziness   ☐ Memory Loss   ☐ Other

Notes

Recommended By:_____

Recommend To:_____

Overall Rating:

☆ ☆ ☆ ☆ ☆

Product

Brand:_____

Name/ Strain:_____

Purchased From:_____

Price:_____

Date Consumed:_____

Current Location:_____

Mood Before Consumption:_____

Mood After Consumption:_____

| Product Type | ☐ Flower | ☐ Edible | ☐ Tincture | ☐ Topical |
| | ☐ Butter/ Oil | ☐ Concentration | ☐ Other | |

| Type | ☐ Sativa | ☐ Indica | ☐ Hybrid |

Terpenes	☐ Pinene	☐ Myrcene	☐ Beta- Caryophyllene
	☐ Limonene	☐ Linalool	☐ Terpinolene
	☐ Humulene	☐ Other	

| Potency mg or % | THC | CBD | CBN | THCA | Other |
| | _____ | _____ | _____ | _____ | _____ |

Method

| ☐ Smoke | ☐ Vaporize | ☐ Vape Pen | ☐ Edible |
| ☐ Drink | ☐ Sublingual | ☐ Capsule | ☐ Patch |

Device:_____

Dose/ # Hits:_____

Taste:_____

My Intent:_____

My Experience

Time Consumed:_____   Time to Kick In:_____

Lasted:_____   Strength: 1 2 3 4 5 6 7 8 9 10

Felt it: Head____%   Body____%   Consume Again: Yes / No

Positive Effects

- Pain Relief
- Stress Reduction
- Anti-Inflammatory
- Energetic
- Muscle Relaxation
- Intestinal Ease
- Creative
- Focused
- Sedative
- Appetite Stimulation
- Anti-Depressant
- Other:

Negative Effects

- Dry Eyes
- Paranoid
- Lethargy
- Anxiety
- Nausea
- Dizziness
- Dry Mouth
- Headache
- Memory Loss
- Confusion
- Drowsy
- Other

Notes

Recommended By:_____

Recommend To:_____

Overall Rating:

☆ ☆ ☆ ☆ ☆

Product

Brand:_____

Name/ Strain:_____

Purchased From:_____

Price:_____

Date Consumed:_____

Current Location:_____

Mood Before Consumption:_____

Mood After Consumption:_____

| **Product Type** | ☐ Flower ☐ Edible ☐ Tincture ☐ Topical |
| | ☐ Butter/ Oil ☐ Concentration ☐ Other |

| **Type** | ☐ Sativa | ☐ Indica | ☐ Hybrid |

| **Terpenes** | ☐ Pinene ☐ Limonene ☐ Humulene | ☐ Myrcene ☐ Linalool ☐ Other | ☐ Beta- Caryophyllene ☐ Terpinolene |

Potency mg or %	THC	CBD	CBN	THCA	Other
	_____	_____	_____	_____	_____

Method

☐ Smoke ☐ Vaporize ☐ Vape Pen ☐ Edible
☐ Drink ☐ Sublingual ☐ Capsule ☐ Patch

Device:_____

Dose/ # Hits:_____

Taste:_____

My Intent:_____

My Experience

Time Consumed:_____   Time to Kick In:_____
Lasted:_____   Strength: 1 2 3 4 5 6 7 8 9 10
Felt it: Head____%   Body____%   Consume Again: Yes / No

Positive Effects

- [ ] Pain Relief
- [ ] Stress Reduction
- [ ] Anti-Inflammatory
- [ ] Energetic
- [ ] Muscle Relaxation
- [ ] Intestinal Ease
- [ ] Creative
- [ ] Focused
- [ ] Sedative
- [ ] Appetite Stimulation
- [ ] Anti-Depressant
- [ ] Other:

Negative Effects

- [ ] Dry Eyes
- [ ] Paranoid
- [ ] Lethargy
- [ ] Anxiety
- [ ] Nausea
- [ ] Dizziness
- [ ] Dry Mouth
- [ ] Headache
- [ ] Memory Loss
- [ ] Confusion
- [ ] Drowsy
- [ ] Other

Notes

Recommended By:

Recommend To:

Overall Rating:

☆ ☆ ☆ ☆ ☆

Product

Brand:_____

Name/ Strain:_____

Purchased From:_____

Price:_____

Date Consumed:_____

Current Location:_____

Mood Before Consumption:_____

Mood After Consumption:_____

| **Product Type** | ☐ Flower | ☐ Edible | ☐ Tincture | ☐ Topical |
| | ☐ Butter/ Oil | ☐ Concentration | ☐ Other | |

| **Type** | ☐ Sativa | ☐ Indica | ☐ Hybrid |

Terpenes	☐ Pinene	☐ Myrcene	☐ Beta- Caryophyllene
	☐ Limonene	☐ Linalool	☐ Terpinolene
	☐ Humulene	☐ Other	

| **Potency mg or %** | THC | CBD | CBN | THCA | Other |
| | _____ | _____ | _____ | _____ | _____ |

Method

| ☐ Smoke | ☐ Vaporize | ☐ Vape Pen | ☐ Edible |
| ☐ Drink | ☐ Sublingual | ☐ Capsule | ☐ Patch |

Device:_____

Dose/ # Hits:_____

Taste:_____

My Intent:_____

My Experience

Time Consumed:_____   Time to Kick In:_____

Lasted:_____   Strength: 1 2 3 4 5 6 7 8 9 10

Felt it: Head____%   Body____%   Consume Again: Yes / No

Positive Effects

- ☐ Pain Relief
- ☐ Stress Reduction
- ☐ Anti-Inflammatory
- ☐ Energetic

- ☐ Muscle Relaxation
- ☐ Intestinal Ease
- ☐ Creative
- ☐ Focused

- ☐ Sedative
- ☐ Appetite Stimulation
- ☐ Anti-Depressant
- ☐ Other:

Negative Effects

- ☐ Dry Eyes
- ☐ Paranoid
- ☐ Lethargy

- ☐ Anxiety
- ☐ Nausea
- ☐ Dizziness

- ☐ Dry Mouth
- ☐ Headache
- ☐ Memory Loss

- ☐ Confusion
- ☐ Drowsy
- ☐ Other

Notes

Recommended By:_____

Recommend To:_____

Overall Rating:

☆ ☆ ☆ ☆ ☆

Product

Brand:_____

Name/ Strain:_____

Purchased From:_____

Price:_____

Date Consumed:_____

Current Location:_____

Mood Before Consumption:_____

Mood After Consumption:_____

| **Product Type** | ☐ Flower | ☐ Edible | ☐ Tincture | ☐ Topical |
| | ☐ Butter/ Oil | ☐ Concentration | ☐ Other | |

| **Type** | ☐ Sativa | ☐ Indica | ☐ Hybrid |

Terpenes	☐ Pinene	☐ Myrcene	☐ Beta- Caryophyllene
	☐ Limonene	☐ Linalool	☐ Terpinolene
	☐ Humulene	☐ Other	

| **Potency mg or %** | THC | CBD | CBN | THCA | Other |
| | _____ | _____ | _____ | _____ | _____ |

Method

☐ Smoke   ☐ Vaporize   ☐ Vape Pen   ☐ Edible
☐ Drink   ☐ Sublingual   ☐ Capsule   ☐ Patch

Device:_____

Dose/ # Hits:_____

Taste:_____

My Intent:_____

My Experience

Time Consumed:_____   Time to Kick In:_____
Lasted:_____   Strength: 1 2 3 4 5 6 7 8 9 10
Felt it: Head____%   Body____%   Consume Again: Yes / No

Positive Effects

☐ Pain Relief   ☐ Muscle Relaxation   ☐ Sedative
☐ Stress Reduction   ☐ Intestinal Ease   ☐ Appetite Stimulation
☐ Anti-Inflammatory   ☐ Creative   ☐ Anti-Depressant
☐ Energetic   ☐ Focused   ☐ Other:

Negative Effects

☐ Dry Eyes   ☐ Anxiety   ☐ Dry Mouth   ☐ Confusion
☐ Paranoid   ☐ Nausea   ☐ Headache   ☐ Drowsy
☐ Lethargy   ☐ Dizziness   ☐ Memory Loss   ☐ Other

Notes
_____
_____
_____
_____
_____
_____
_____
_____

Recommended By: Overall Rating:
_____
                                         ☆ ☆ ☆ ☆ ☆
Recommend To:
_____

Product

Brand:_____

Name/ Strain:_____

Purchased From:_____

Price:_____

Date Consumed:_____

Current Location:_____

Mood Before Consumption:_____

Mood After Consumption:_____

| **Product Type** | ☐ Flower | ☐ Edible | ☐ Tincture | ☐ Topical |
| | ☐ Butter/ Oil | ☐ Concentration | ☐ Other | |

| **Type** | ☐ Sativa | ☐ Indica | ☐ Hybrid |

Terpenes	☐ Pinene	☐ Myrcene	☐ Beta- Caryophyllene
	☐ Limonene	☐ Linalool	☐ Terpinolene
	☐ Humulene	☐ Other	

| **Potency mg or %** | THC | CBD | CBN | THCA | Other |
| | _____ | _____ | _____ | _____ | _____ |

Method

| ☐ Smoke | ☐ Vaporize | ☐ Vape Pen | ☐ Edible |
| ☐ Drink | ☐ Sublingual | ☐ Capsule | ☐ Patch |

Device:_____

Dose/ # Hits:_____

Taste:_____

My Intent:_____

My Experience

Time Consumed:_____   Time to Kick In:_____
Lasted:___·_____   Strength: 1 2 3 4 5 6 7 8 9 10
Felt it: Head___% Body___%   Consume Again: Yes / No

Positive Effects

- [ ] Pain Relief
- [ ] Stress Reduction
- [ ] Anti-Inflammatory
- [ ] Energetic

- [ ] Muscle Relaxation
- [ ] Intestinal Ease
- [ ] Creative
- [ ] Focused

- [ ] Sedative
- [ ] Appetite Stimulation
- [ ] Anti-Depressant
- [ ] Other:

Negative Effects

- [ ] Dry Eyes
- [ ] Paranoid
- [ ] Lethargy

- [ ] Anxiety
- [ ] Nausea
- [ ] Dizziness

- [ ] Dry Mouth
- [ ] Headache
- [ ] Memory Loss

- [ ] Confusion
- [ ] Drowsy
- [ ] Other

Notes

_____
_____
_____
_____
_____
_____
_____
_____

Recommended By: _____

Recommend To: _____

Overall Rating: _____

☆ ☆ ☆ ☆ ☆

Product

Brand:_____

Name/ Strain:_____

Purchased From:_____

Price:_____

Date Consumed:_____

Current Location:_____

Mood Before Consumption:_____

Mood After Consumption:_____

Product Type	☐ Flower ☐ Butter/ Oil	☐ Edible ☐ Concentration	☐ Tincture ☐ Other	☐ Topical
Type	☐ Sativa	☐ Indica	☐ Hybrid	
Terpenes	☐ Pinene ☐ Limonene ☐ Humulene	☐ Myrcene ☐ Linalool ☐ Other	☐ Beta- Caryophyllene ☐ Terpinolene	

Potency mg or %	THC	CBD	CBN	THCA	Other
	_____	_____	_____	_____	_____

Method

☐ Smoke   ☐ Vaporize   ☐ Vape Pen   ☐ Edible
☐ Drink   ☐ Sublingual   ☐ Capsule   ☐ Patch

Device:_____

Dose/ # Hits:_____

Taste:_____

My Intent:_____

My Experience

Time Consumed:_____   Time to Kick In:_____
Lasted:_____   Strength: 1 2 3 4 5 6 7 8 9 10
Felt it: Head___% Body___%   Consume Again: Yes / No

Positive Effects

☐ Pain Relief   ☐ Muscle Relaxation   ☐ Sedative
☐ Stress Reduction   ☐ Intestinal Ease   ☐ Appetite Stimulation
☐ Anti-Inflammatory   ☐ Creative   ☐ Anti-Depressant
☐ Energetic   ☐ Focused   ☐ Other:

Negative Effects

☐ Dry Eyes   ☐ Anxiety   ☐ Dry Mouth   ☐ Confusion
☐ Paranoid   ☐ Nausea   ☐ Headache   ☐ Drowsy
☐ Lethargy   ☐ Dizziness   ☐ Memory Loss   ☐ Other

Notes

Recommended By:_____

Recommend To:_____

Overall Rating:

☆ ☆ ☆ ☆ ☆

Product

Brand:_____

Name/ Strain:_____

Purchased From:_____

Price:_____

Date Consumed:_____

Current Location:_____

Mood Before Consumption:_____

Mood After Consumption:_____

Product Type	☐ Flower	☐ Edible	☐ Tincture	☐ Topical
	☐ Butter/ Oil	☐ Concentration	☐ Other	

Type	☐ Sativa	☐ Indica	☐ Hybrid

Terpenes	☐ Pinene	☐ Myrcene	☐ Beta- Caryophyllene
	☐ Limonene	☐ Linalool	☐ Terpinolene
	☐ Humulene	☐ Other	

Potency mg or %	THC	CBD	CBN	THCA	Other
	_____	_____	_____	_____	_____

Method

☐ Smoke ☐ Vaporize ☐ Vape Pen ☐ Edible
☐ Drink ☐ Sublingual ☐ Capsule ☐ Patch

Device:_____

Dose/ # Hits:_____

Taste:_____

My Intent:_____

My Experience

Time Consumed:_____ Time to Kick In:_____
Lasted:_____ Strength: 1 2 3 4 5 6 7 8 9 10
Felt it: Head___% Body___% Consume Again: Yes / No

Positive Effects

☐ Pain Relief ☐ Muscle Relaxation ☐ Sedative
☐ Stress Reduction ☐ Intestinal Ease ☐ Appetite Stimulation
☐ Anti-Inflammatory ☐ Creative ☐ Anti-Depressant
☐ Energetic ☐ Focused ☐ Other:

Negative Effects

☐ Dry Eyes ☐ Anxiety ☐ Dry Mouth ☐ Confusion
☐ Paranoid ☐ Nausea ☐ Headache ☐ Drowsy
☐ Lethargy ☐ Dizziness ☐ Memory Loss ☐ Other

Notes

Recommended By: Overall Rating:
_____

Recommend To:
_____ ☆ ☆ ☆ ☆ ☆

Product

Brand:_____

Name/ Strain:_____

Purchased From:_____

Price:_____

Date Consumed:_____

Current Location:_____

Mood Before Consumption:_____

Mood After Consumption:_____

| **Product Type** | ☐ Flower | ☐ Edible | ☐ Tincture | ☐ Topical |
| | ☐ Butter/ Oil | ☐ Concentration | ☐ Other | |

| **Type** | ☐ Sativa | ☐ Indica | ☐ Hybrid |

Terpenes	☐ Pinene	☐ Myrcene	☐ Beta- Caryophyllene
	☐ Limonene	☐ Linalool	☐ Terpinolene
	☐ Humulene	☐ Other	

| **Potency mg or %** | THC | CBD | CBN | THCA | Other |
| | _____ | _____ | _____ | _____ | _____ |

Method

| ☐ Smoke | ☐ Vaporize | ☐ Vape Pen | ☐ Edible |
| ☐ Drink | ☐ Sublingual | ☐ Capsule | ☐ Patch |

Device:_____

Dose/ # Hits:_____

Taste:_____

My Intent:_____

My Experience

Time Consumed:_____ Time to Kick In:_____

Lasted:_____ Strength: 1 2 3 4 5 6 7 8 9 10

Felt it: Head____% Body____% Consume Again: Yes / No

Positive Effects

☐ Pain Relief ☐ Muscle Relaxation ☐ Sedative
☐ Stress Reduction ☐ Intestinal Ease ☐ Appetite Stimulation
☐ Anti-Inflammatory ☐ Creative ☐ Anti-Depressant
☐ Energetic ☐ Focused ☐ Other:

Negative Effects

☐ Dry Eyes ☐ Anxiety ☐ Dry Mouth ☐ Confusion
☐ Paranoid ☐ Nausea ☐ Headache ☐ Drowsy
☐ Lethargy ☐ Dizziness ☐ Memory Loss ☐ Other

Notes

Recommended By:_____

Recommend To:_____

Overall Rating:

☆ ☆ ☆ ☆ ☆

Product

Brand:_____

Name/ Strain:_____

Purchased From:_____

Price:_____

Date Consumed:_____

Current Location:_____

Mood Before Consumption:_____

Mood After Consumption:_____

Product Type	☐ Flower ☐ Edible ☐ Tincture ☐ Topical ☐ Butter/ Oil ☐ Concentration ☐ Other
Type	☐ Sativa ☐ Indica ☐ Hybrid
Terpenes	☐ Pinene ☐ Myrcene ☐ Beta- Caryophyllene ☐ Limonene ☐ Linalool ☐ Terpinolene ☐ Humulene ☐ Other

Potency mg or %	THC	CBD	CBN	THCA	Other
	_____	_____	_____	_____	_____

Method

☐ Smoke   ☐ Vaporize   ☐ Vape Pen   ☐ Edible
☐ Drink   ☐ Sublingual   ☐ Capsule   ☐ Patch

Device:_____

Dose/ # Hits:_____

Taste:_____

My Intent:_____

My Experience

Time Consumed:_____ Time to Kick In:_____

Lasted:_____ Strength: 1 2 3 4 5 6 7 8 9 10

Felt it: Head____% Body____% Consume Again: Yes / No

Positive Effects

- ☐ Pain Relief
- ☐ Stress Reduction
- ☐ Anti-Inflammatory
- ☐ Energetic

- ☐ Muscle Relaxation
- ☐ Intestinal Ease
- ☐ Creative
- ☐ Focused

- ☐ Sedative
- ☐ Appetite Stimulation
- ☐ Anti-Depressant
- ☐ Other:

Negative Effects

- ☐ Dry Eyes
- ☐ Paranoid
- ☐ Lethargy

- ☐ Anxiety
- ☐ Nausea
- ☐ Dizziness

- ☐ Dry Mouth
- ☐ Headache
- ☐ Memory Loss

- ☐ Confusion
- ☐ Drowsy
- ☐ Other

Notes

Recommended By:_____

Recommend To:_____

Overall Rating:

☆ ☆ ☆ ☆ ☆

Product

Brand:_____

Name/ Strain:_____

Purchased From:_____

Price:_____

Date Consumed:_____

Current Location:_____

Mood Before Consumption:_____

Mood After Consumption:_____

Product Type	☐ Flower ☐ Butter/ Oil	☐ Edible ☐ Concentration	☐ Tincture ☐ Other	☐ Topical

Type	☐ Sativa	☐ Indica	☐ Hybrid

Terpenes	☐ Pinene ☐ Limonene ☐ Humulene	☐ Myrcene ☐ Linalool ☐ Other	☐ Beta- Caryophyllene ☐ Terpinolene

Potency mg or %	THC	CBD	CBN	THCA	Other
	_____	_____	_____	_____	_____

Method

☐ Smoke   ☐ Vaporize   ☐ Vape Pen   ☐ Edible
☐ Drink   ☐ Sublingual   ☐ Capsule   ☐ Patch

Device:_____

Dose/ # Hits:_____

Taste:_____

My Intent:_____

My Experience

Time Consumed:_____   Time to Kick In:_____
Lasted:_____   Strength: 1 2 3 4 5 6 7 8 9 10
Felt it: Head____% Body____%   Consume Again: Yes / No

Positive Effects

☐ Pain Relief   ☐ Muscle Relaxation   ☐ Sedative
☐ Stress Reduction   ☐ Intestinal Ease   ☐ Appetite Stimulation
☐ Anti-Inflammatory   ☐ Creative   ☐ Anti-Depressant
☐ Energetic   ☐ Focused   ☐ Other:

Negative Effects

☐ Dry Eyes   ☐ Anxiety   ☐ Dry Mouth   ☐ Confusion
☐ Paranoid   ☐ Nausea   ☐ Headache   ☐ Drowsy
☐ Lethargy   ☐ Dizziness   ☐ Memory Loss   ☐ Other

Notes

Recommended By: _____   Overall Rating:

Recommend To: _____   ☆ ☆ ☆ ☆ ☆

Product

Brand:_____

Name/ Strain:_____

Purchased From:_____

Price:_____

Date Consumed:_____

Current Location:_____

Mood Before Consumption:_____

Mood After Consumption:_____

Product Type	☐ Flower	☐ Edible	☐ Tincture	☐ Topical
	☐ Butter/ Oil	☐ Concentration	☐ Other	

Type	☐ Sativa	☐ Indica	☐ Hybrid

Terpenes	☐ Pinene	☐ Myrcene	☐ Beta- Caryophyllene
	☐ Limonene	☐ Linalool	☐ Terpinolene
	☐ Humulene	☐ Other	

Potency mg or %	THC	CBD	CBN	THCA	Other
	_____	_____	_____	_____	_____

Method

☐ Smoke	☐ Vaporize	☐ Vape Pen	☐ Edible
☐ Drink	☐ Sublingual	☐ Capsule	☐ Patch

Device:_____

Dose/ # Hits:_____

Taste:_____

My Intent:_____

My Experience

Time Consumed:_____   Time to Kick In:_____

Lasted:_____   Strength: 1 2 3 4 5 6 7 8 9 10

Felt it: Head____% Body____%   Consume Again: Yes / No

Positive Effects

☐ Pain Relief   ☐ Muscle Relaxation   ☐ Sedative
☐ Stress Reduction   ☐ Intestinal Ease   ☐ Appetite Stimulation
☐ Anti-Inflammatory   ☐ Creative   ☐ Anti-Depressant
☐ Energetic   ☐ Focused   ☐ Other:

Negative Effects

☐ Dry Eyes   ☐ Anxiety   ☐ Dry Mouth   ☐ Confusion
☐ Paranoid   ☐ Nausea   ☐ Headache   ☐ Drowsy
☐ Lethargy   ☐ Dizziness   ☐ Memory Loss   ☐ Other

Notes

Recommended By:_____

Recommend To:_____

Overall Rating:

☆ ☆ ☆ ☆ ☆

Product

Brand:_____

Name/ Strain:_____

Purchased From:_____

Price:_____

Date Consumed:_____

Current Location:_____

Mood Before Consumption:_____

Mood After Consumption:_____

Product Type	☐ Flower	☐ Edible	☐ Tincture	☐ Topical
	☐ Butter/ Oil	☐ Concentration	☐ Other	

Type	☐ Sativa	☐ Indica	☐ Hybrid

Terpenes	☐ Pinene	☐ Myrcene	☐ Beta- Caryophyllene
	☐ Limonene	☐ Linalool	☐ Terpinolene
	☐ Humulene	☐ Other	

Potency mg or %	THC	CBD	CBN	THCA	Other
	_____	_____	_____	_____	_____

Method

☐ Smoke	☐ Vaporize	☐ Vape Pen	☐ Edible
☐ Drink	☐ Sublingual	☐ Capsule	☐ Patch

Device:_____

Dose/ # Hits:_____

Taste:_____

My Intent:_____

My Experience

Time Consumed:_____   Time to Kick In:_____

Lasted:_____   Strength: 1 2 3 4 5 6 7 8 9 10

Felt it: Head____%   Body____%   Consume Again: Yes / No

Positive Effects

☐ Pain Relief   ☐ Muscle Relaxation   ☐ Sedative
☐ Stress Reduction   ☐ Intestinal Ease   ☐ Appetite Stimulation
☐ Anti-Inflammatory   ☐ Creative   ☐ Anti-Depressant
☐ Energetic   ☐ Focused   ☐ Other:

Negative Effects

☐ Dry Eyes   ☐ Anxiety   ☐ Dry Mouth   ☐ Confusion
☐ Paranoid   ☐ Nausea   ☐ Headache   ☐ Drowsy
☐ Lethargy   ☐ Dizziness   ☐ Memory Loss   ☐ Other

Notes

Recommended By:

Recommend To:

Overall Rating:

☆ ☆ ☆ ☆ ☆

Product

Brand:_____

Name/ Strain:_____

Purchased From:_____

Price:_____

Date Consumed:_____

Current Location:_____

Mood Before Consumption:_____

Mood After Consumption:_____

Product Type	☐ Flower ☐ Butter/ Oil	☐ Edible ☐ Concentration	☐ Tincture ☐ Other	☐ Topical
Type	☐ Sativa	☐ Indica	☐ Hybrid	
Terpenes	☐ Pinene ☐ Limonene ☐ Humulene	☐ Myrcene ☐ Linalool ☐ Other	☐ Beta- Caryophyllene ☐ Terpinolene	

Potency mg or %	THC	CBD	CBN	THCA	Other
	_____	_____	_____	_____	_____

Method

☐ Smoke   ☐ Vaporize   ☐ Vape Pen   ☐ Edible
☐ Drink   ☐ Sublingual   ☐ Capsule   ☐ Patch

Device:_____

Dose/ # Hits:_____

Taste:_____

My Intent:_____

My Experience

Time Consumed:_____   Time to Kick In:_____

Lasted:_____   Strength: 1 2 3 4 5 6 7 8 9 10

Felt it: Head____% Body____%   Consume Again: Yes / No

Positive Effects

- ☐ Pain Relief
- ☐ Stress Reduction
- ☐ Anti-Inflammatory
- ☐ Energetic

- ☐ Muscle Relaxation
- ☐ Intestinal Ease
- ☐ Creative
- ☐ Focused

- ☐ Sedative
- ☐ Appetite Stimulation
- ☐ Anti-Depressant
- ☐ Other:

Negative Effects

- ☐ Dry Eyes
- ☐ Paranoid
- ☐ Lethargy

- ☐ Anxiety
- ☐ Nausea
- ☐ Dizziness

- ☐ Dry Mouth
- ☐ Headache
- ☐ Memory Loss

- ☐ Confusion
- ☐ Drowsy
- ☐ Other

Notes

Recommended By:_____

Recommend To:_____

Overall Rating:

☆ ☆ ☆ ☆ ☆

Product

Brand:_____

Name/ Strain:_____

Purchased From:_____

Price:_____

Date Consumed:_____

Current Location:_____

Mood Before Consumption:_____

Mood After Consumption:_____

Product Type	☐ Flower	☐ Edible	☐ Tincture	☐ Topical
	☐ Butter/ Oil	☐ Concentration	☐ Other	

Type	☐ Sativa	☐ Indica	☐ Hybrid

Terpenes	☐ Pinene	☐ Myrcene	☐ Beta- Caryophyllene
	☐ Limonene	☐ Linalool	☐ Terpinolene
	☐ Humulene	☐ Other	

Potency mg or %	THC	CBD	CBN	THCA	Other
	_____	_____	_____	_____	_____

Method

☐ Smoke	☐ Vaporize	☐ Vape Pen	☐ Edible
☐ Drink	☐ Sublingual	☐ Capsule	☐ Patch

Device:_____

Dose/ # Hits:_____

Taste:_____

My Intent:_____

My Experience

Time Consumed:_____ Time to Kick In:_____

Lasted:_____ Strength: 1 2 3 4 5 6 7 8 9 10

Felt it: Head___% Body___% Consume Again: Yes / No

Positive Effects

- [ ] Pain Relief
- [ ] Stress Reduction
- [ ] Anti-Inflammatory
- [ ] Energetic
- [ ] Muscle Relaxation
- [ ] Intestinal Ease
- [ ] Creative
- [ ] Focused
- [ ] Sedative
- [ ] Appetite Stimulation
- [ ] Anti-Depressant
- [ ] Other:

Negative Effects

- [ ] Dry Eyes
- [ ] Paranoid
- [ ] Lethargy
- [ ] Anxiety
- [ ] Nausea
- [ ] Dizziness
- [ ] Dry Mouth
- [ ] Headache
- [ ] Memory Loss
- [ ] Confusion
- [ ] Drowsy
- [ ] Other

Notes

Recommended By: _____

Recommend To: _____

Overall Rating:

☆ ☆ ☆ ☆ ☆

Product

Brand:_____

Name/ Strain:_____

Purchased From:_____

Price:_____

Date Consumed:_____

Current Location:_____

Mood Before Consumption:_____

Mood After Consumption:_____

Product Type	☐ Flower ☐ Butter/ Oil	☐ Edible ☐ Concentration	☐ Tincture ☐ Other	☐ Topical

Type	☐ Sativa	☐ Indica	☐ Hybrid

Terpenes	☐ Pinene ☐ Limonene ☐ Humulene	☐ Myrcene ☐ Linalool ☐ Other	☐ Beta- Caryophyllene ☐ Terpinolene

Potency mg or %	THC	CBD	CBN	THCA	Other
	_____	_____	_____	_____	_____

Method

☐ Smoke ☐ Vaporize ☐ Vape Pen ☐ Edible
☐ Drink ☐ Sublingual ☐ Capsule ☐ Patch

Device:_____

Dose/ # Hits:_____

Taste:_____

My Intent:_____

My Experience

Time Consumed:_____   Time to Kick In:_____
Lasted:_____   Strength: 1 2 3 4 5 6 7 8 9 10
Felt it: Head____% Body____%   Consume Again: Yes / No

Positive Effects

☐ Pain Relief   ☐ Muscle Relaxation   ☐ Sedative
☐ Stress Reduction   ☐ Intestinal Ease   ☐ Appetite Stimulation
☐ Anti-Inflammatory   ☐ Creative   ☐ Anti-Depressant
☐ Energetic   ☐ Focused   ☐ Other:

Negative Effects

☐ Dry Eyes   ☐ Anxiety   ☐ Dry Mouth   ☐ Confusion
☐ Paranoid   ☐ Nausea   ☐ Headache   ☐ Drowsy
☐ Lethargy   ☐ Dizziness   ☐ Memory Loss   ☐ Other

Notes

Recommended By: Overall Rating:

Recommend To: ☆ ☆ ☆ ☆ ☆

Product

Brand:_____

Name/ Strain:_____

Purchased From:_____

Price:_____

Date Consumed:_____

Current Location:_____

Mood Before Consumption:_____

Mood After Consumption:_____

Product Type	☐ Flower ☐ Butter/ Oil	☐ Edible ☐ Concentration	☐ Tincture ☐ Other	☐ Topical

Type	☐ Sativa	☐ Indica	☐ Hybrid

Terpenes	☐ Pinene ☐ Limonene ☐ Humulene	☐ Myrcene ☐ Linalool ☐ Other	☐ Beta- Caryophyllene ☐ Terpinolene

Potency mg or %	THC	CBD	CBN	THCA	Other
	_____	_____	_____	_____	_____

Method

☐ Smoke   ☐ Vaporize   ☐ Vape Pen   ☐ Edible
☐ Drink   ☐ Sublingual   ☐ Capsule   ☐ Patch

Device:_____

Dose/ # Hits:_____

Taste:_____

My Intent:_____

My Experience

Time Consumed:_____   Time to Kick In:_____

Lasted:_____   Strength: 1 2 3 4 5 6 7 8 9 10

Felt it: Head____% Body____%   Consume Again: Yes / No

Positive Effects

☐ Pain Relief   ☐ Muscle Relaxation   ☐ Sedative
☐ Stress Reduction   ☐ Intestinal Ease   ☐ Appetite Stimulation
☐ Anti-Inflammatory ☐ Creative   ☐ Anti-Depressant
☐ Energetic   ☐ Focused   ☐ Other:

Negative Effects

☐ Dry Eyes   ☐ Anxiety   ☐ Dry Mouth   ☐ Confusion
☐ Paranoid   ☐ Nausea   ☐ Headache   ☐ Drowsy
☐ Lethargy   ☐ Dizziness   ☐ Memory Loss   ☐ Other

Notes

_____
_____
_____
_____
_____
_____
_____
_____

Recommended By: Overall Rating:
_____

Recommend To: ☆ ☆ ☆ ☆ ☆
_____

Product

Brand:_____

Name/ Strain:_____

Purchased From:_____

Price:_____

Date Consumed:_____

Current Location:_____

Mood Before Consumption:_____

Mood After Consumption:_____

| **Product Type** | ☐ Flower | ☐ Edible | ☐ Tincture | ☐ Topical |
| | ☐ Butter/ Oil | ☐ Concentration | ☐ Other | |

| **Type** | ☐ Sativa | ☐ Indica | ☐ Hybrid |

Terpenes	☐ Pinene	☐ Myrcene	☐ Beta- Caryophyllene
	☐ Limonene	☐ Linalool	☐ Terpinolene
	☐ Humulene	☐ Other	

| **Potency mg or %** | THC | CBD | CBN | THCA | Other |
| | _____ | _____ | _____ | _____ | _____ |

Method

| ☐ Smoke | ☐ Vaporize | ☐ Vape Pen | ☐ Edible |
| ☐ Drink | ☐ Sublingual | ☐ Capsule | ☐ Patch |

Device:_____

Dose/ # Hits:_____

Taste:_____

My Intent:_____

My Experience

Time Consumed:_____ Time to Kick In:_____
Lasted:_____ Strength: 1 2 3 4 5 6 7 8 9 10
Felt it: Head____% Body____%   Consume Again: Yes / No

Positive Effects

☐ Pain Relief   ☐ Muscle Relaxation   ☐ Sedative
☐ Stress Reduction   ☐ Intestinal Ease   ☐ Appetite Stimulation
☐ Anti-Inflammatory   ☐ Creative   ☐ Anti-Depressant
☐ Energetic   ☐ Focused   ☐ Other:

Negative Effects

☐ Dry Eyes   ☐ Anxiety   ☐ Dry Mouth   ☐ Confusion
☐ Paranoid   ☐ Nausea   ☐ Headache   ☐ Drowsy
☐ Lethargy   ☐ Dizziness   ☐ Memory Loss   ☐ Other

Notes

Recommended By:

Recommend To:

Overall Rating:

☆ ☆ ☆ ☆ ☆

Product

Brand:_____

Name/ Strain:_____

Purchased From:_____

Price:_____

Date Consumed:_____

Current Location:_____

Mood Before Consumption:_____

Mood After Consumption:_____

Product Type	☐ Flower ☐ Butter/ Oil	☐ Edible ☐ Concentration	☐ Tincture ☐ Other	☐ Topical

Type	☐ Sativa	☐ Indica	☐ Hybrid

Terpenes	☐ Pinene ☐ Limonene ☐ Humulene	☐ Myrcene ☐ Linalool ☐ Other	☐ Beta- Caryophyllene ☐ Terpinolene

Potency mg or %	THC	CBD	CBN	THCA	Other
	_____	_____	_____	_____	_____

Method

☐ Smoke   ☐ Vaporize   ☐ Vape Pen   ☐ Edible
☐ Drink   ☐ Sublingual   ☐ Capsule   ☐ Patch

Device:_____

Dose/ # Hits:_____

Taste:_____

My Intent:_____

My Experience

Time Consumed:_____   Time to Kick In:_____
Lasted:_____   Strength: 1 2 3 4 5 6 7 8 9 10
Felt it: Head____% Body____%   Consume Again: Yes / No

Positive Effects

☐ Pain Relief   ☐ Muscle Relaxation   ☐ Sedative
☐ Stress Reduction   ☐ Intestinal Ease   ☐ Appetite Stimulation
☐ Anti-Inflammatory   ☐ Creative   ☐ Anti-Depressant
☐ Energetic   ☐ Focused   ☐ Other:

Negative Effects

☐ Dry Eyes   ☐ Anxiety   ☐ Dry Mouth   ☐ Confusion
☐ Paranoid   ☐ Nausea   ☐ Headache   ☐ Drowsy
☐ Lethargy   ☐ Dizziness   ☐ Memory Loss   ☐ Other

Notes

Recommended By:

Recommend To:

Overall Rating:

☆ ☆ ☆ ☆ ☆

Product

Brand:_____

Name/ Strain:_____

Purchased From:_____

Price:_____

Date Consumed:_____

Current Location:_____

Mood Before Consumption:_____

Mood After Consumption:_____

| **Product Type** | ☐ Flower | ☐ Edible | ☐ Tincture | ☐ Topical |
| | ☐ Butter/ Oil | ☐ Concentration | ☐ Other | |

| **Type** | ☐ Sativa | ☐ Indica | ☐ Hybrid |

Terpenes	☐ Pinene	☐ Myrcene	☐ Beta- Caryophyllene
	☐ Limonene	☐ Linalool	☐ Terpinolene
	☐ Humulene	☐ Other	

| **Potency mg or %** | THC | CBD | CBN | THCA | Other |
| | _____ | _____ | _____ | _____ | _____ |

Method

| ☐ Smoke | ☐ Vaporize | ☐ Vape Pen | ☐ Edible |
| ☐ Drink | ☐ Sublingual | ☐ Capsule | ☐ Patch |

Device:_____

Dose/ # Hits:_____

Taste:_____

My Intent:_____

My Experience

Time Consumed:_____ Time to Kick In:_____

Lasted:_____ Strength: 1 2 3 4 5 6 7 8 9 10

Felt it: Head___% Body___% Consume Again: Yes / No

Positive Effects

- ☐ Pain Relief
- ☐ Stress Reduction
- ☐ Anti-Inflammatory
- ☐ Energetic
- ☐ Muscle Relaxation
- ☐ Intestinal Ease
- ☐ Creative
- ☐ Focused
- ☐ Sedative
- ☐ Appetite Stimulation
- ☐ Anti-Depressant
- ☐ Other:

Negative Effects

- ☐ Dry Eyes
- ☐ Paranoid
- ☐ Lethargy
- ☐ Anxiety
- ☐ Nausea
- ☐ Dizziness
- ☐ Dry Mouth
- ☐ Headache
- ☐ Memory Loss
- ☐ Confusion
- ☐ Drowsy
- ☐ Other

Notes

Recommended By:_____

Recommend To:_____

Overall Rating:

☆ ☆ ☆ ☆ ☆

Product

Brand:_____

Name/ Strain:_____

Purchased From:_____

Price:_____

Date Consumed:_____

Current Location:_____

Mood Before Consumption:_____

Mood After Consumption:_____

Product Type	☐ Flower	☐ Edible	☐ Tincture	☐ Topical
	☐ Butter/ Oil	☐ Concentration	☐ Other	

Type	☐ Sativa	☐ Indica	☐ Hybrid

Terpenes	☐ Pinene	☐ Myrcene	☐ Beta- Caryophyllene
	☐ Limonene	☐ Linalool	☐ Terpinolene
	☐ Humulene	☐ Other	

Potency mg or %	THC	CBD	CBN	THCA	Other
	_____	_____	_____	_____	_____

Method

☐ Smoke	☐ Vaporize	☐ Vape Pen	☐ Edible
☐ Drink	☐ Sublingual	☐ Capsule	☐ Patch

Device:_____

Dose/ # Hits:_____

Taste:_____

My Intent:_____

My Experience

Time Consumed:_____   Time to Kick In:_____
Lasted:_____   Strength: 1 2 3 4 5 6 7 8 9 10
Felt it: Head____% Body____%   Consume Again: Yes / No

Positive Effects

- Pain Relief
- Stress Reduction
- Anti-Inflammatory
- Energetic

- Muscle Relaxation
- Intestinal Ease
- Creative
- Focused

- Sedative
- Appetite Stimulation
- Anti-Depressant
- Other:

Negative Effects

- Dry Eyes
- Paranoid
- Lethargy

- Anxiety
- Nausea
- Dizziness

- Dry Mouth
- Headache
- Memory Loss

- Confusion
- Drowsy
- Other

Notes

Recommended By:

Recommend To:

Overall Rating:

☆ ☆ ☆ ☆ ☆

Product

Brand:_____

Name/ Strain:_____

Purchased From:_____

Price:_____

Date Consumed:_____

Current Location:_____

Mood Before Consumption:_____

Mood After Consumption:_____

Product Type	☐ Flower ☐ Butter/ Oil	☐ Edible ☐ Concentration	☐ Tincture ☐ Other	☐ Topical

Type	☐ Sativa	☐ Indica	☐ Hybrid

Terpenes	☐ Pinene ☐ Limonene ☐ Humulene	☐ Myrcene ☐ Linalool ☐ Other	☐ Beta- Caryophyllene ☐ Terpinolene

Potency mg or %	THC	CBD	CBN	THCA	Other
	_____	_____	_____	_____	_____

Method

☐ Smoke	☐ Vaporize	☐ Vape Pen	☐ Edible
☐ Drink	☐ Sublingual	☐ Capsule	☐ Patch

Device:_____

Dose/ # Hits:_____

Taste:_____

My Intent:_____

My Experience

Time Consumed:_____ Time to Kick In:_____
Lasted:_____ Strength: 1 2 3 4 5 6 7 8 9 10
Felt it: Head___% Body___% Consume Again: Yes / No

Positive Effects

☐ Pain Relief   ☐ Muscle Relaxation   ☐ Sedative
☐ Stress Reduction   ☐ Intestinal Ease   ☐ Appetite Stimulation
☐ Anti-Inflammatory   ☐ Creative   ☐ Anti-Depressant
☐ Energetic   ☐ Focused   ☐ Other:

Negative Effects

☐ Dry Eyes   ☐ Anxiety   ☐ Dry Mouth   ☐ Confusion
☐ Paranoid   ☐ Nausea   ☐ Headache   ☐ Drowsy
☐ Lethargy   ☐ Dizziness   ☐ Memory Loss   ☐ Other

Notes

Recommended By: _____

Recommend To: _____

Overall Rating:

☆ ☆ ☆ ☆ ☆

Product

Brand:_____

Name/ Strain:_____

Purchased From:_____

Price:_____

Date Consumed:_____

Current Location:_____

Mood Before Consumption:_____

Mood After Consumption:_____

Product Type	☐ Flower ☐ Butter/ Oil	☐ Edible ☐ Concentration	☐ Tincture ☐ Other	☐ Topical

Type	☐ Sativa	☐ Indica	☐ Hybrid

Terpenes	☐ Pinene ☐ Limonene ☐ Humulene	☐ Myrcene ☐ Linalool ☐ Other	☐ Beta- Caryophyllene ☐ Terpinolene

Potency mg or %	THC	CBD	CBN	THCA	Other
	_____	_____	_____	_____	_____

Method

☐ Smoke   ☐ Vaporize   ☐ Vape Pen   ☐ Edible
☐ Drink   ☐ Sublingual   ☐ Capsule   ☐ Patch

Device:_____

Dose/ # Hits:_____

Taste:_____

My Intent:_____

My Experience

Time Consumed:_____   Time to Kick In:_____
Lasted:_____   Strength: 1 2 3 4 5 6 7 8 9 10
Felt it: Head____% Body____%   Consume Again: Yes / No

Positive Effects

- [ ] Pain Relief
- [ ] Stress Reduction
- [ ] Anti-Inflammatory
- [ ] Energetic
- [ ] Muscle Relaxation
- [ ] Intestinal Ease
- [ ] Creative
- [ ] Focused
- [ ] Sedative
- [ ] Appetite Stimulation
- [ ] Anti-Depressant
- [ ] Other:

Negative Effects

- [ ] Dry Eyes
- [ ] Paranoid
- [ ] Lethargy
- [ ] Anxiety
- [ ] Nausea
- [ ] Dizziness
- [ ] Dry Mouth
- [ ] Headache
- [ ] Memory Loss
- [ ] Confusion
- [ ] Drowsy
- [ ] Other

Notes

Recommended By: Overall Rating:

Recommend To: ☆ ☆ ☆ ☆ ☆

Product

Brand:_____

Name/ Strain:_____

Purchased From:_____

Price:_____

Date Consumed:_____

Current Location:_____

Mood Before Consumption:_____

Mood After Consumption:_____

| Product Type | ☐ Flower | ☐ Edible | ☐ Tincture | ☐ Topical |
| | ☐ Butter/ Oil | ☐ Concentration | ☐ Other | |

| Type | ☐ Sativa | ☐ Indica | ☐ Hybrid |

Terpenes	☐ Pinene	☐ Myrcene	☐ Beta- Caryophyllene
	☐ Limonene	☐ Linalool	☐ Terpinolene
	☐ Humulene	☐ Other	

| Potency mg or % | THC | CBD | CBN | THCA | Other |
| | _____ | _____ | _____ | _____ | _____ |

Method

| ☐ Smoke | ☐ Vaporize | ☐ Vape Pen | ☐ Edible |
| ☐ Drink | ☐ Sublingual | ☐ Capsule | ☐ Patch |

Device:_____

Dose/ # Hits:_____

Taste:_____

My Intent:_____

My Experience

Time Consumed:_____ Time to Kick In:_____

Lasted:_____ Strength: 1 2 3 4 5 6 7 8 9 10

Felt it: Head___% Body___% Consume Again: Yes / No

Positive Effects

- ☐ Pain Relief
- ☐ Stress Reduction
- ☐ Anti-Inflammatory
- ☐ Energetic

- ☐ Muscle Relaxation
- ☐ Intestinal Ease
- ☐ Creative
- ☐ Focused

- ☐ Sedative
- ☐ Appetite Stimulation
- ☐ Anti-Depressant
- ☐ Other:

Negative Effects

- ☐ Dry Eyes
- ☐ Paranoid
- ☐ Lethargy

- ☐ Anxiety
- ☐ Nausea
- ☐ Dizziness

- ☐ Dry Mouth
- ☐ Headache
- ☐ Memory Loss

- ☐ Confusion
- ☐ Drowsy
- ☐ Other

Notes

Recommended By:

Recommend To:

Overall Rating:

☆ ☆ ☆ ☆ ☆

Product

Brand:_____

Name/ Strain:_____

Purchased From:_____

Price:_____ . _____

Date Consumed:_____

Current Location:_____

Mood Before Consumption:_____

Mood After Consumption:_____

Product Type	☐ Flower ☐ Butter/ Oil	☐ Edible ☐ Concentration	☐ Tincture ☐ Other	☐ Topical

Type	☐ Sativa	☐ Indica	☐ Hybrid

Terpenes	☐ Pinene ☐ Limonene ☐ Humulene	☐ Myrcene ☐ Linalool ☐ Other	☐ Beta- Caryophyllene ☐ Terpinolene

Potency mg or %	THC	CBD	CBN	THCA	Other
	_____	_____	_____	_____	_____

Method

☐ Smoke   ☐ Vaporize   ☐ Vape Pen   ☐ Edible
☐ Drink   ☐ Sublingual   ☐ Capsule   ☐ Patch

Device:_____

Dose/ # Hits:_____

Taste:_____

My Intent:_____

My Experience

Time Consumed:_____   Time to Kick In:_____

Lasted:_____   Strength: 1 2 3 4 5 6 7 8 9 10

Felt it: Head____%   Body____%   Consume Again: Yes / No

Positive Effects

- [ ] Pain Relief
- [ ] Stress Reduction
- [ ] Anti-Inflammatory
- [ ] Energetic

- [ ] Muscle Relaxation
- [ ] Intestinal Ease
- [ ] Creative
- [ ] Focused

- [ ] Sedative
- [ ] Appetite Stimulation
- [ ] Anti-Depressant
- [ ] Other:

Negative Effects

- [ ] Dry Eyes
- [ ] Paranoid
- [ ] Lethargy

- [ ] Anxiety
- [ ] Nausea
- [ ] Dizziness

- [ ] Dry Mouth
- [ ] Headache
- [ ] Memory Loss

- [ ] Confusion
- [ ] Drowsy
- [ ] Other

Notes

Recommended By:

Recommend To:

Overall Rating:

☆☆☆☆☆

Product

Brand:_____

Name/ Strain:_____

Purchased From:_____

Price:_____

Date Consumed:_____

Current Location:_____

Mood Before Consumption:_____

Mood After Consumption:_____

| **Product Type** | ☐ Flower | ☐ Edible | ☐ Tincture | ☐ Topical |
| | ☐ Butter/ Oil | ☐ Concentration | ☐ Other | |

| **Type** | ☐ Sativa | ☐ Indica | ☐ Hybrid |

Terpenes	☐ Pinene	☐ Myrcene	☐ Beta- Caryophyllene
	☐ Limonene	☐ Linalool	☐ Terpinolene
	☐ Humulene	☐ Other	

| **Potency mg or %** | THC | CBD | CBN | THCA | Other |
| | _____ | _____ | _____ | _____ | _____ |

Method

| ☐ Smoke | ☐ Vaporize | ☐ Vape Pen | ☐ Edible |
| ☐ Drink | ☐ Sublingual | ☐ Capsule | ☐ Patch |

Device:_____

Dose/ # Hits:_____

Taste:_____

My Intent:_____

My Experience

Time Consumed:_____   Time to Kick In:_____
Lasted:_____   Strength: 1 2 3 4 5 6 7 8 9 10
Felt it: Head____% Body____%   Consume Again: Yes / No

Positive Effects

☐ Pain Relief   ☐ Muscle Relaxation   ☐ Sedative
☐ Stress Reduction   ☐ Intestinal Ease   ☐ Appetite Stimulation
☐ Anti-Inflammatory   ☐ Creative   ☐ Anti-Depressant
☐ Energetic   ☐ Focused   ☐ Other:

Negative Effects

☐ Dry Eyes   ☐ Anxiety   ☐ Dry Mouth   ☐ Confusion
☐ Paranoid   ☐ Nausea   ☐ Headache   ☐ Drowsy
☐ Lethargy   ☐ Dizziness   ☐ Memory Loss   ☐ Other

Notes

_____
_____
_____
_____
_____
_____
_____

Recommended By: _____   Overall Rating:

Recommend To: _____   ☆ ☆ ☆ ☆ ☆

Product

Brand:_____

Name/ Strain:_____

Purchased From:_____

Price:_____

Date Consumed:_____

Current Location:_____

Mood Before Consumption:_____

Mood After Consumption:_____

| Product Type | ☐ Flower ☐ Edible ☐ Tincture ☐ Topical |
| | ☐ Butter/ Oil ☐ Concentration ☐ Other |

| Type | ☐ Sativa | ☐ Indica | ☐ Hybrid |

Terpenes	☐ Pinene	☐ Myrcene	☐ Beta- Caryophyllene
	☐ Limonene	☐ Linalool	☐ Terpinolene
	☐ Humulene	☐ Other	

Potency mg or %	THC	CBD	CBN	THCA	Other
	_____	_____	_____	_____	_____

Method

☐ Smoke   ☐ Vaporize   ☐ Vape Pen   ☐ Edible
☐ Drink   ☐ Sublingual   ☐ Capsule   ☐ Patch

Device:_____

Dose/ # Hits:_____

Taste:_____

My Intent:_____

My Experience

Time Consumed:_____   Time to Kick In:_____
Lasted:_____   Strength: 1 2 3 4 5 6 7 8 9 10
Felt it: Head____%   Body____%   Consume Again: Yes / No

Positive Effects

☐ Pain Relief   ☐ Muscle Relaxation   ☐ Sedative
☐ Stress Reduction   ☐ Intestinal Ease   ☐ Appetite Stimulation
☐ Anti-Inflammatory   ☐ Creative   ☐ Anti-Depressant
☐ Energetic   ☐ Focused   ☐ Other:

Negative Effects

☐ Dry Eyes   ☐ Anxiety   ☐ Dry Mouth   ☐ Confusion
☐ Paranoid   ☐ Nausea   ☐ Headache   ☐ Drowsy
☐ Lethargy   ☐ Dizziness   ☐ Memory Loss   ☐ Other

Notes

Recommended By:

Recommend To:

Overall Rating:

☆ ☆ ☆ ☆ ☆

Product

Brand:_____

Name/ Strain:_____

Purchased From:_____

Price:_____

Date Consumed:_____

Current Location:_____

Mood Before Consumption:_____

Mood After Consumption:_____

Product Type	☐ Flower ☐ Butter/ Oil	☐ Edible ☐ Concentration	☐ Tincture ☐ Other	☐ Topical

Type	☐ Sativa	☐ Indica	☐ Hybrid

Terpenes	☐ Pinene ☐ Limonene ☐ Humulene	☐ Myrcene ☐ Linalool ☐ Other	☐ Beta- Caryophyllene ☐ Terpinolene

Potency mg or %	THC	CBD	CBN	THCA	Other
	_____	_____	_____	_____	_____

Method

☐ Smoke ☐ Vaporize ☐ Vape Pen ☐ Edible
☐ Drink ☐ Sublingual ☐ Capsule ☐ Patch

Device:_____

Dose/ # Hits:_____

Taste:_____

My Intent:_____

My Experience

Time Consumed:_____ Time to Kick In:_____
Lasted:_____ Strength: 1 2 3 4 5 6 7 8 9 10
Felt it: Head___% Body___% Consume Again: Yes / No

Positive Effects

☐ Pain Relief   ☐ Muscle Relaxation   ☐ Sedative
☐ Stress Reduction   ☐ Intestinal Ease   ☐ Appetite Stimulation
☐ Anti-Inflammatory   ☐ Creative   ☐ Anti-Depressant
☐ Energetic   ☐ Focused   ☐ Other:

Negative Effects

☐ Dry Eyes   ☐ Anxiety   ☐ Dry Mouth   ☐ Confusion
☐ Paranoid   ☐ Nausea   ☐ Headache   ☐ Drowsy
☐ Lethargy   ☐ Dizziness   ☐ Memory Loss   ☐ Other

Notes

_____
_____
_____
_____
_____
_____
_____
_____
_____

Recommended By: _____

Recommend To: _____

Overall Rating:

☆ ☆ ☆ ☆ ☆

Product

Brand:_____

Name/ Strain:_____

Purchased From:_____

Price:_____

Date Consumed:_____

Current Location:_____

Mood Before Consumption:_____

Mood After Consumption:_____

Product Type	☐ Flower ☐ Butter/ Oil	☐ Edible ☐ Concentration	☐ Tincture ☐ Other	☐ Topical

Type	☐ Sativa	☐ Indica	☐ Hybrid

Terpenes	☐ Pinene ☐ Limonene ☐ Humulene	☐ Myrcene ☐ Linalool ☐ Other	☐ Beta- Caryophyllene ☐ Terpinolene

Potency mg or %	THC	CBD	CBN	THCA	Other
	_____	_____	_____	_____	_____

Method

☐ Smoke   ☐ Vaporize   ☐ Vape Pen   ☐ Edible
☐ Drink   ☐ Sublingual   ☐ Capsule   ☐ Patch

Device:_____

Dose/ # Hits:_____

Taste:_____

My Intent:_____

My Experience

Time Consumed:_____   Time to Kick In:_____

Lasted:_____   Strength: 1 2 3 4 5 6 7 8 9 10

Felt it: Head___%   Body___%   Consume Again: Yes / No

Positive Effects

☐ Pain Relief   ☐ Muscle Relaxation   ☐ Sedative
☐ Stress Reduction   ☐ Intestinal Ease   ☐ Appetite Stimulation
☐ Anti-Inflammatory   ☐ Creative   ☐ Anti-Depressant
☐ Energetic   ☐ Focused   ☐ Other:

Negative Effects

☐ Dry Eyes   ☐ Anxiety   ☐ Dry Mouth   ☐ Confusion
☐ Paranoid   ☐ Nausea   ☐ Headache   ☐ Drowsy
☐ Lethargy   ☐ Dizziness   ☐ Memory Loss   ☐ Other

Notes

Recommended By: Overall Rating:

Recommend To: ☆ ☆ ☆ ☆ ☆

Made in United States
Troutdale, OR
03/27/2024